CW00500111

The Complete KETO Chaffle Cooking Guide

Amazing Chaffle Recipes For Weight Loss

Lily Sherman

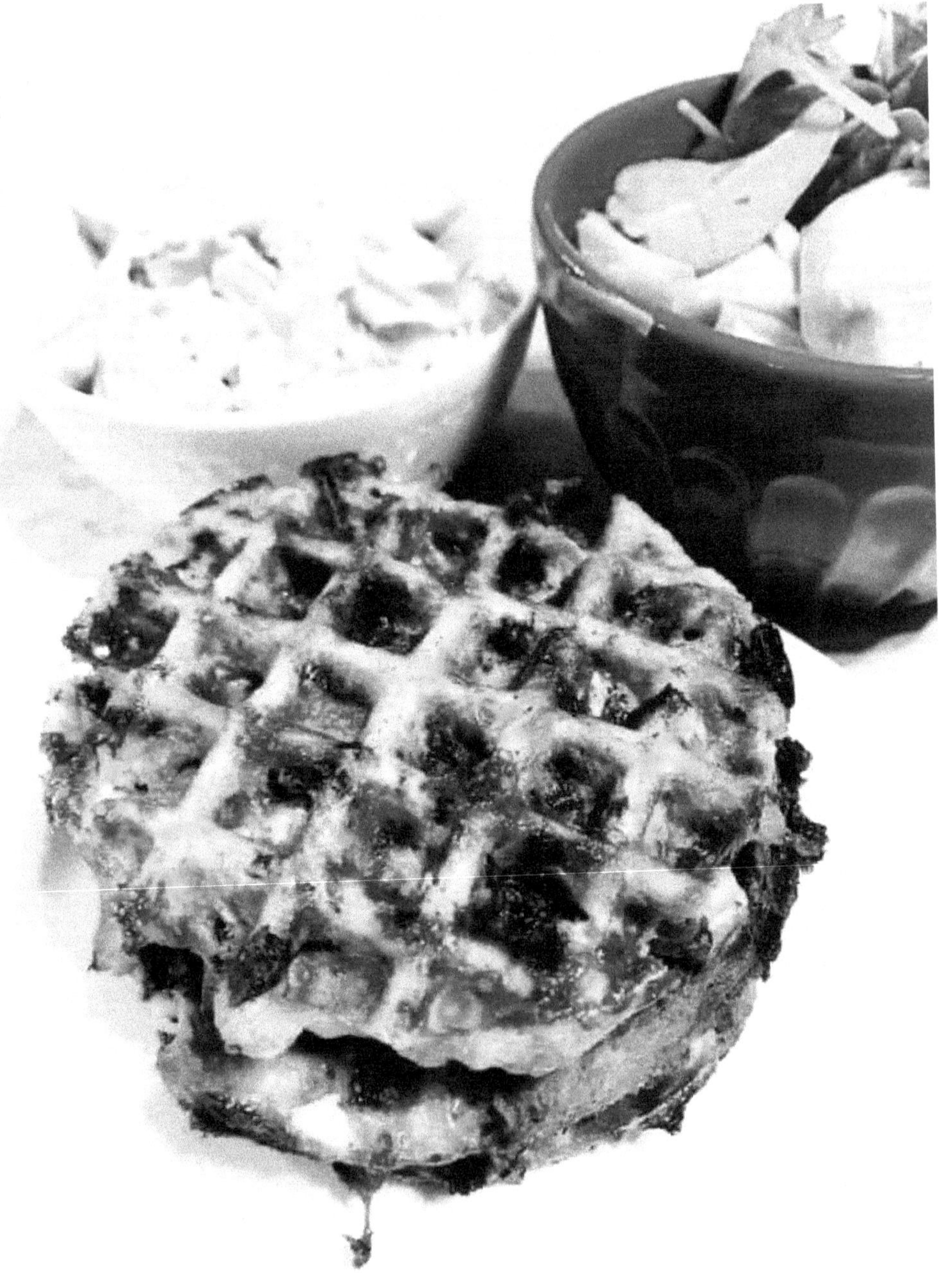

Table of contents

Sour Cream Protein Chaffles

Cooking: 16 Minutes

Servings: 4

Ingredients

- 6 organic eggs
- 1/2 cup sour cream
- 1/2 cup unsweetened whey protein powder
- 1 teaspn organic baking powder
- 1/2 teaspn salt
- 1 cup Cheddar cheese, shredded

Directions

1. Preheat now a waffle iron and then grease it.
2. In a bowl, place all ingredients and Mix well until well combined.
3. Place 1/4 of the mixture into Preheat nowed waffle iron and cook for about 4 minutes or until golden brown.
4. Repeat now with the remaining mixture.
5. Serve warm.

Nutrition:

Net Carb: 3g, Fat: 22.6g, Saturated Fat: 11.9g, Carbohydrates: 3.6g, Sugar: 1.3 g, Protein: 27.3g

Jicama Hash Brown Chaffle

Preparation: 15-20 minutes

Servings: 4

Ingredients

- 1 large jicama root
- 1/2 medium onion minced
- 2 garlic cloves pressed
- 1 cup cheese of choice I used Halloumi
- 2 eggs whisked
- Salt and Pepper

Directions

1. Peel jicama
2. Shred in food processor
3. Place shredded jicama in large colander, sprinkle with 1-2 tsp of salt. Mix well and allow to drain.
4. Squeeze out as much liquid as possible (very important step)
5. Microwave for 5-8 minutes
6. Mix all Ingredients

7. Sprinkle a little cheese on waffle iron before adding 3 T of mixture, sprinkle a little more cheese

Nutrition:

Total Fat: 11.8g 15%, Cholesterol: 121 mg 40%, Sodium: 221.8 mg 10%, Total Carbohydrate: 5.1 g 2%, Dietary Fiber: 1.7 g 6%, Sugars: 1.2 g, Protein 10 g 20%, Vitamin A: 133.5µg 15%, Vitamin C: 7.3 mg 8%

Egg on A Cheddar Cheese Chaffle

Cooking: 7–9 Minutes

Servings: 4

Ingredients

Batter:

- 4 eggs
- 2 cups shredded white cheddar cheese
- Salt and pepper to taste

Other:

- 2 tbsps butter for brushing your waffle maker
- 4 large eggs
- 2 tbsps olive oil

Directions

1. Preheat now your waffle maker.
2. Crack the eggs into a bowl and whisk them with a fork.
3. Stir in the grated cheddar cheese and season with salt and pepper.

4. Brush the heated waffle maker with butter and add a few tbsps of the batter. Close the lid and cook for about 7–8 minutes depending on your waffle maker.
5. While chaffles are cooking, cook the eggs.
6. Warm the oil in a large non-stick pan with a lid over medium-low heat for 2-3 minutes.
7. Crack an egg in a tiny ramekin and gently add it to the pan.
8. Repeat the same way for the other 3 eggs.
9. Cover and let cook for 2 to 2 ½ minutes for set eggs but with runny yolks.
10. Remove now from heat. To serve, place a chaffle on each plate and top with an egg.
11. Season with salt and black pepper to taste.

Nutrition:

Calories: 4, Fat: 34 g, Carbs: 2 g, Sugar: 0.6 g, Protein: 26 g, Sodium: 518 mg

Avocado Chaffle Toast

Cooking: 10 Minutes

Servings: 3

Ingredients

- 4 tbsps. avocado mash
- 1/2 tsp lemon juice
- 1/8 tsp salt
- 1/8 tsp black pepper
- 2 eggs
- 1/2 cup shredded cheese

For Servings:

- 3 eggs
- ½ avocado thinly sliced
- 1 tomato, sliced

Directions

1. Mash avocado mash with lemon juice, salt, and black pepper in mixing bowl, until well combined.
2. In a tiny bowl beat egg and pour eggs in avocado mixture and mix well.

3. Switch on Waffle Maker to pre-heat.
4. Pour 1/8 of shredded cheese in a waffle maker and then pour ½ of egg and avocado mixture and then 1/8 shredded cheese.
5. Close the lid and cook chaffles for about 3 - 4 minutes.
6. Repeat now with the remaining mixture.
7. Meanwhile, fry eggs in a pan for about 1-2 minutes.
8. For serving, arrange fried egg on chaffle toast with avocado slice and tomatoes. Sprinkle salt and pepper on top and enjoy!

Nutrition:

Protein: 26% 66 kcal, Fat: 67% 169 kcal, Carbohydrates: 6% 15 kcal

Cajun & Feta Chaffles

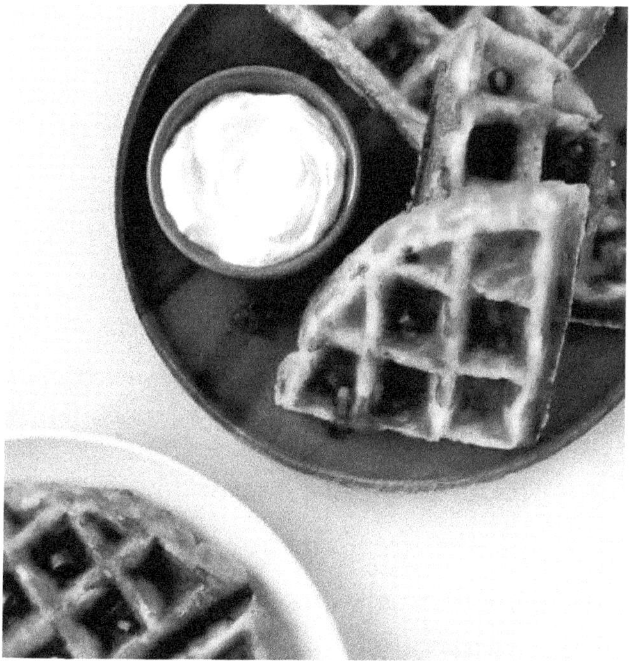

Cooking: 10 Minutes

Servings: 1

Ingredients

- 1 egg white
- 1/4 cup shredded mozzarella cheese
- 2 tbsps. almond flour

- 1 tsp Cajun Seasoning

For Serving:

- 1 egg
- 4 oz. feta cheese
- 1 tomato, sliced

Directions

1. Whisk together egg, cheese, and seasoning in a bowl.
2. Switch on and grease waffle maker with cooking spray.
3. Pour batter in a Preheat nowed waffle maker.
4. Cook chaffles for about 2-3 minutes until the chaffle is cooked through.
5. Meanwhile, fry the egg in a non-stick pan for about 1-2 minutes.
6. For serving set fried egg on chaffles with feta cheese and tomatoes slice.

Nutrition:

Protein: 28% 119 kcal, Fat: 64% 2 kcal, Carbohydrates: 7% 31 kcal

Taco Chaffle (Indicare Pagina)

Cooking: 20 Minutes

Servings: 4

Ingredients

- 1 tbspn olive oil
- 1 lb. ground beef
- 1 teaspn ground cumin
- 1 teaspn chili powder
- 1/4 teaspn onion powder
- 1/2 teaspn garlic powder
- Salt to taste
- 4 basic chaffles
- 1 cup cabbage, chopped
- 4 tbsps salsa (sugar-free)

Directions

1. Pour the olive oil into a pan over medium heat.
2. Add the ground beef.
3. Season with the salt and spices.
4. Cook until brown and crumbly.

5. Fold the chaffle to create a "taco shell".
6. Stuff each chaffle taco with cabbage.
7. Top with the ground beef and salsa.

Nutrition:

Calories: 255, Saturated Fat: 3.2g, Cholesterol: 10mg, Sodium: 220mg, Potassium: 561mg, Total Carbohydrate: 39, Protein: 35.1g, Total Sugars: 1g.

Maple Chaffle

Cooking: 15 Minutes

Servings: 2

Ingredients

- 1 egg, lightly beaten
- 2 egg whites
- 1/2 tsp maple extract
- 2 tsp Swerve
- 1/2 tsp baking powder, gluten-free
- 2 tbsp almond milk
- 2 tbsp coconut flour

Directions

1. Preheat now your waffle maker.
2. In a bowl, whip egg whites until stiff peaks form.
3. Stir in maple extract, Swerve, baking powder, almond milk, coconut flour, and egg.
4. Spray waffle maker with cooking spray.

5. Pour half batter in the hot waffle maker and cook for 3-minutes or until golden brown. Repeat now with the remaining batter.
6. Serve and enjoy.

Nutrition:

Calories: 122, Fat: 6.6 g, Carbohydrates: 9 g, Sugar: 1 g, Protein: 7 g, Cholesterol: 82 mg

Egg & Avocado Chaffle Sandwich

Cooking: 10 Minutes

Servings: 2

Ingredients

- Cooking spray
- 4 slices bacon
- 2 eggs
- 1/2 avocado, mashed
- 4 basic chaffles
- 2 leaves lettuce

Directions

1. Coat your skillet with cooking spray.
2. Cook the bacon until golden and crisp.
3. Transfer into a paper towel lined plate.
4. Crack the eggs into the same pan and cook until firm.
5. Flip and cook until the yolk is set.
6. Spread the avocado on the chaffle.
7. Top with lettuce, egg and bacon.
8. Top with another chaffle.

Nutrition:

Calories 372, Total Fat 30.1g, Saturated Fat 8.6g, Cholesterol 205mg, Total Carbohydrate 5.49g, Dietary Fiber 3.49g, Total Sugars 0.6g, Protein20.6g, Potassium 524mg

Sausage & Egg Chaffle Sandwich

Cooking: 10 Minutes

Servings: 1

Ingredients

- 2 basics cooked chaffles
- 1 tbspn olive oil
- 1 sausage, sliced into rounds
- 1 egg

Directions

1. Pour olive oil into your pan over medium heat.
2. Put it over medium heat.
3. Add the sausage and cook until brown on both sides.
4. Put the sausage rounds on top of one chaffle.
5. Cook the egg in the same pan without mixing.
6. Place on top of the sausage rounds.
7. Top with another chaffle.

Nutrition:

Calories 332, Total Fat 21.6g, Saturated Fat 4.49, Cholesterol 139mg, Potassium 16g, Sodium 463mg, Total Carbohydrate 24.9g, Dietary Fiber 0g, Protein 10g, Total Sugars 0.2g

Bacon Chaffle For Singles

Cooking: 8 Minutes

Servings: 1

Ingredients

- 1 egg
- 1/2 cup Swiss cheese
- 2 tbsps cooked crumbled bacon

Directions

1. Preheat now your waffle maker.
2. Beat the egg in a bowl.
3. Stir in the cheese and bacon.
4. Pour half of the mixture into the device.
5. Close and cook for 4 minutes.
6. Cook the second chaffle using the same steps.

Nutrition:

Calories 23, Total Fat 17.6g, Saturated Fat 8.1g, Cholesterol 128mg, Sodium 522mg, Dietary Fiber 0g, Total Sugars 0.5g, Protein 17.1g, Potassium 158mg

Bacon & Egg Chaffles

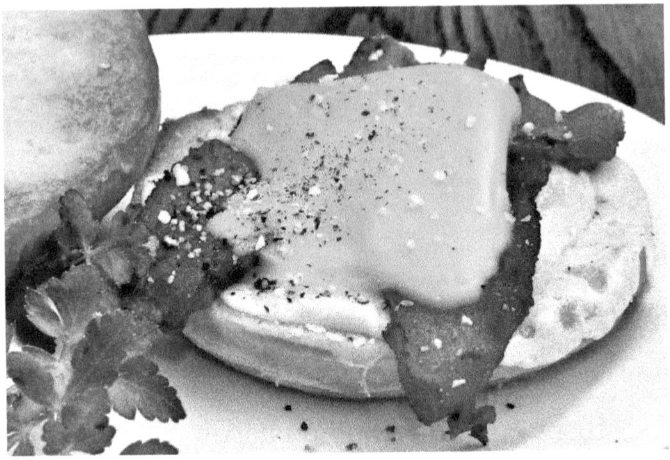

Cooking: 10 Minutes

Servings: 2

Ingredients

- 2 eggs
- 4 tsp collagen peptides, grass-fed
- 2 tbsp pork panko
- 3 slices crispy bacon

Directions

1. Warm up your mini waffle maker.

2. Combine the eggs, pork panko, and collagen peptides. Mix well. Divide the batter in two tiny bowls.
3. Once done, evenly distribute 1/2 of the crispy chopped bacon on your waffle maker.
4. Pour one bowl of the batter over the bacon. cook for 5 minutes and immediately repeat this step for the second chaffle.
5. Plate your cooked chaffles and sprinkle with extra Panko for an added crunch
6. Enjoy!

Nutrition:

Calories per Servings**:** 266 Kcal; Fats: 1g ; Carbs: 11.2 g ; Protein: 27 g

Sausage Chaffles

Cooking: 10-15 min

Servings: 1-2

Ingredients

- 1 pound gluten-free bulk Italian sausage crumbled
- 1 organic egg, beaten
- 1 cup sharp Cheddar cheese, shredded
- 1/4 cup Parmesan cheese, grated
- 1 cup almond flour
- 2 teaspns organic baking powder

Directions

1. Preheat now a mini waffle iron and then grease It.
2. In a bowl, place all ingredients and Mix well until well combined with your hands.
3. Place about 3 tbsps of the mixture 1 into Preheat nowed waffle iron and cook for about 3 minutes or until golden brown.
4. Carefully, flip the chaffle and cook for about 2 minutes or until golden brown.

5. Repeat now with the remaining mixture.
6. Serve warm.

Nutrition:

Calories: 238, Net Carb: 1 .2 g, Fat: 1 9.6 g, Saturated Fat: 6.1g, Carbohydrates: 2.2g, Dietary Fiber: 1g, Sugar 0.4g, Protein 10.8g

Egg & Chives Chaffle Sandwich Roll

Cooking: 10 Minute

Servings: 2

Ingredients

- 2 tbsps mayonnaise
- 1 hard-boiled egg, chopped
- 1 tbspn chives, chopped
- 2 basic chaffles

Directions:

1. In a bowl, mix now the mayo, egg and chives.
2. Spread the mixture on top of the chaffles.
3. Roll the chaffle.

Nutrition:

Calories 258, Total Fat 12g, Saturated Fat 2.8g, Cholesterol 171mg, Sodium 271mg, Potassium 71mg, Total Carbohydrate 7.5g, Dietary Fiber 0.1g, Protein 5.9g, Total Sugars 2.3g

Crispy Chaffles With Sausage

Cooking: 10 Minutes

Servings: 2

Ingredients

- 1/2 cup cheddar cheese
- 1/2 tsp. baking powder
- 1/4 cup egg whites
- 2 tsp. pumpkin spice

<u>For Serving:</u>

- 1 egg, whole
- 2 chicken sausage
- 2 slice bacon
- salt and pepper to taste
- 1 tsp. avocado oil

Directions

1. Mix all ingredients in a bowl.
2. Allow batter to sit while waffle iron warms.
3. Spray waffle iron with nonstick spray.

4. Pour batter in your waffle maker and cook according to the manufacturer's directions.
5. Meanwhile, heat oil in a pan and fry the egg, according to your choice and transfer it to a plate. In the same pan, fry bacon slice and sausage on medium heat for about 2-3 minutes until cooked.
6. Once chaffles are cooked thoroughly, Remove now them from the maker.
7. Serve with fried egg, bacon slice, sausages and enjoy!

Nutrition:

Protein: 22% 86 kcal, Fat: 74% 286 kcal, Carbohydrates: 3% 12 kcal

Chaffle Tortilla

Cooking: 8 Minutes

Servings: 2

Ingredients

- 1 egg
- 1/2 cup cheddar cheese, shredded
- 1 teaspn baking powder
- 4 tbsps almond flour
- 1/4 teaspn garlic powder
- 1 tbspn almond milk
- Homemade salsa
- Sour cream
- Jalapeno pepper, chopped

Directions

1. Preheat now your waffle maker.
2. Beat the egg in a bowl.
3. Stir in the cheese, baking powder, flour, garlic powder and almond milk.
4. Pour half of the batter into your waffle maker.
5. Cover and cook for 4 minutes.

6. Open and transfer to a plate. Let cool for 2 minutes.
7. Do the same for the remaining batter.
8. Top the waffle with salsa, sour cream and jalapeno pepper.
9. Roll the waffle.

Nutrition:

Calories 225, Total Fat 17.6g, Saturated Fat 9.99g, Sodium 367mg, Potassium 366mg, Total Carbohydrate 6g, Dietary Fiber 0.8g, Protein 11.3g, Total Sugars 1.9g

Mixed Berry & Vanilla Chaffles

Preparation: 10 minutes

Cooking: 28 minutes

Servings: 4

Ingredients

- 1 egg, beaten
- ½ cup finely grated mozzarella cheese
- 1 tbsp cream cheese, softened
- 1 tbsp sugar-free maple syrup
- 2 strawberries, sliced
- 2 raspberries, slices
- ¼ tsp blackberry extract
- ¼ tsp vanilla extract
- ½ cup plain yogurt for serving

Directions

1. Preheat now the waffle iron.
2. In a bowl, mix all the ingredients except the yogurt.
3. Open the iron, lightly grease with cooking spray and pour in a quarter of the mixture.

4. Close the iron and cook until golden brown and crispy, 7 minutes.
5. Remove now the chaffle onto a plate and set aside.
6. Make three more chaffles with the remaining mixture.
7. To serve: top with the yogurt and enjoy.

Nutrition:

Calories: 99 Cal, Total Fat: 8 g, Șaturated Fat: 0 g, Cholesterol: 0 mg, Sodium: 0 mg, Total Carbs: 4 g

Chicken Quesadilla Chaffle

Preparation: 10 minutes

Cooking: 14 minutes

Servings: 2

Ingredients

- 1 egg, beaten
- ¼ tsp taco seasoning
- 1/3 cup of finely grated cheddar cheese
- 1/3 cup of cooked chopped chicken

Directions

1. Preheat now the waffle iron.
2. In a bowl, mix now the egg, taco seasoning, and cheddar cheese. Add the chicken and combine well.
3. Open the iron, lightly grease with cooking spray and pour in half of the mixture.
4. Close the iron and cook until brown and crispy, 7 minutes.
5. Remove now the chaffle onto a plate and set aside.
6. Make another chaffle using the remaining mixture.

7. Serve afterward.

Nutrition:

Calories: 99 Cal, Total Fat: 8 g, Saturated Fat: 0 g, Cholesterol: 0 mg, Sodium: 0 mg, Total Carbs: 4 g

Hot Chocolate Breakfast Chaffle

Preparation: 15 minutes

Cooking: 14 Minutes

Servings: 2

Ingredients

- 1 egg, beaten
- 2 tbsp. almond flour
- 1 tbsp. unsweetened cocoa powder
- 2 tbsp. cream cheese, softened
- ¼ cup finely grated Monterey Jack cheese
- 2 tbsp. sugar-free maple syrup
- 1 tsp. vanilla extract

Directions

1. Preheat now the waffle iron.
2. In a bowl, mix all the ingredients.
3. Open the iron, lightly grease with cooking spray and pour in half of the mixture.
4. Close the iron and cooking until crispy, 7 minutes.
5. Remove now the chaffle onto a plate and set aside.

6. Pour the remaining batter in the iron and make the second chaffle.
7. Allow cooling and serve afterward.

Nutrition:

Calories: 203, Protein: 19 g, Fats: 10 g, Carbohydrates: 5 g

Delicious Raspberries Chaffles

Preparation: 20 min

Cooking: 15 min

Servings: 1

Ingredients

- 1 egg white
- 1/4 cup jack cheese, shredded
- 1/4 cup cheddar cheese, shredded
- 1 tsp. coconut flour
- 1/4 tsp. baking powder
- 1/2 tsp. stevia

<u>For Topping:</u>

- 4 oz. raspberries
- 2 tbsps. coconut flour
- 2 oz. unsweetened raspberry sauce

Directions

1. Switch on your round Waffle Maker and grease it with cooking spray once hot.

2. Mix all chaffle ingredients in a bowl and combine with a fork.
3. Pour chaffle batter in a Preheat nowed maker and close the lid.
4. Roll the taco chaffle around using a kitchen roller, set it aside and allow it to set for a few minutes.
5. Once the taco chaffle is set, Remove now from the roller.
6. Dip raspberries in sauce and arrange on taco chaffle.
7. Drizzle coconut flour on top.
8. Enjoy raspberries taco chaffle with keto coffee.

Nutrition:

Calories: 54, Protein: 3 g, Fat: 4.1 g, Carbohydrates: 1.1 g

Japanese Styled Chaffle

Preparation: 12 minutes

Cooking: 6 minutes

Servings: 2

Ingredients

- Egg: 1
- Bacon: 1 slice
- Green onion: 1 stalk
- Mozzarella cheese: 1/2 cup (shredded)
- Kewpie Mayo: 2 tbsps

Directions

- Preheat now and grease your waffle maker. Using a mixing bowl, a mix containing kewpie mayo with beaten egg, then add in ½ chopped green onion with the other ½ kept aside, and ¼ inches of cut bacon into the mixture.
- Mix evenly. Sprinkle your waffle maker's base with 1/8 cup of shredded Mozzarella and pour in the mixture, then top with more shredded mozzarella.

With a closed lid, heat the waffle for 5 minutes to a crunch and then Remove now the chaffle and allow cooking for a few minutes.

- Repeat for the remaining chaffles mixture to make more batter. Serve by garnishing the chaffle with the leftover chopped green onions. Enjoy.

Nutrition:

Calories 92 Kcal Fat: 7 g Protein: 1 g Net carb: 2 g

Keto Strawberry Chaffle

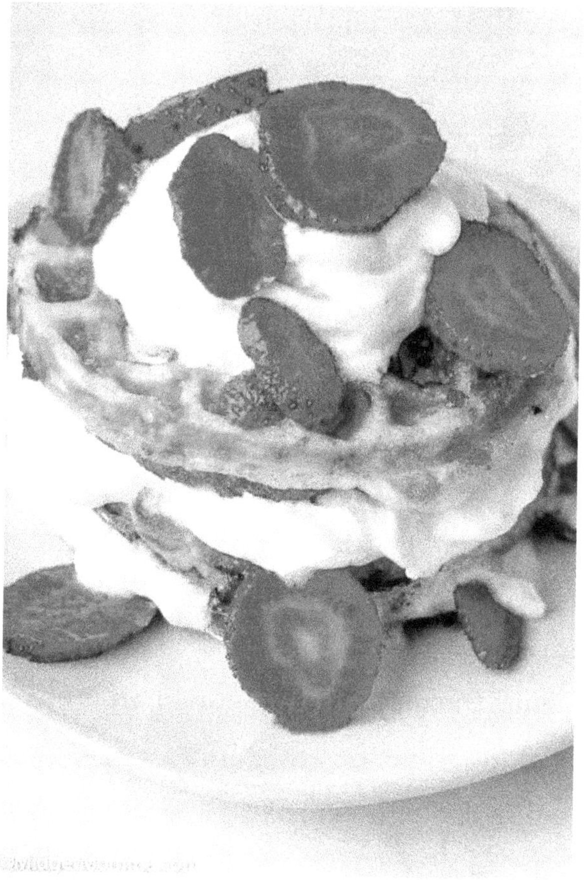

Preparation: 10 minutes

Cooking: 5 minutes

Servings: 2

Ingredients

- 1 egg
- 1/4 cup Mozzarella cheese
- 1 tbspnful cream cheese
- 1/4 teaspnful baking powder
- 2 sliced strawberries
- 1 teaspnful strawberry extract

Directions

- Preheat now waffle maker.
- In a little bowl, beat the egg.
- Add the rest of the ingredients.
- Your waffle maker is sprayed with nonstick cooking spray.
- Divide the mix into two equal parts.
- Cooking a portion of the mix for around 4 minutes or until golden brown colored.

Nutrition:

Calories: 249, Fat: 20g, Carbs: 3g, Protein: 15g

Keto Crunchy Chaffle

Preparation: 15 minutes

Cooking: 8 minutes

Servings: 2

Ingredients

- 2 Large Eggs
- 1/2 Cup Shredded Mozzarella cheese (pressed firmly)
- 1/2 teaspn Baking Powder
- 1 Tbspn Erythritol (powder), or sweetener (however powder is most ideal)
- 1/2 teaspn Vanilla Extract

Directions:

- Heat You Waffle Iron on the high heat setting
- Put all ingredients into a Bullet or a Blender and blend for 10 seconds.
- Pour the mix into a very hot and dry waffle Iron. It will look thin once poured but have no fear it significantly increases in size when cooking (and you'll need to keep an eye on it to avoid overflow

when cooking!). Let the waffle to Cooking for 3-4 minutes or much more! The waffle is done once the entire waffle is golden dark-colored, which takes longer than a normal waffle would. You can use a fork to flip your waffle to ensure that each side has even colors if it doesn't look done after some time. Let waffle cool for 3-4 minutes before eating since it may become brown on cooling

- Serve with gobs of grass-fed butter and sugar-free syrup, or whatever topping you want.

Nutrition:

Calories: 155, Fat: 14g, Protein: 5g, Net Carbs: 2g

Keto Silver Dollar Pancakes

Preparation: 10 minutes

Cooking: 5 minutes

Servings: 2

Ingredients

- (3) Eggs
- 1/2 Cup (105 G) Cottage Cheese
- 1/3 cup of (37.33 G) Superfine Almond Flour
- 1/4 Cup (62.5 G) Unsweetened Almond Milk
- 2 Tbsps Truvia
- Vanilla Extract
- 1 Teaspn Baking Powder
- Cooking Oil Spray

Directions

- Place ingredients in a blender in the order listed above. Mix well until you have a smooth, fluid batter.
- Heat a nonstick pan on medium-high temperature. Spray with oil or margarine.
- Place 2 tbsps of batter at once to make little, dollar hotcakes. This is an extremely fluid, sensitive batter

so don't attempt to make big pancakes with this one as they won't flip over easily.

- Cooking every pancake until the top of the hotcake has made little air pockets and the air pockets have vanished, around 1-2 minutes.
- Using a spatula, tenderly loosen the pan cake, and afterward flip over.
- Make the remainder of the pancakes and serve hot.

Nutrition:

Calories: 110, Fat: 8g, Protein: 2g, Net Carbs: 7g

Keto Chaffle Waffle

Preparation: 10 minutes

Cooking: 6 minutes

Servings: 2

Ingredients

- 1 egg
- ½ cup of shredded Mozzarella cheese
- 1 ½ table-spoon of almond flour
- Pinch of baking powder

Directions

1. Start by turning your waffle maker on and Preheat nowing it. During pre-heating, in a bowl, whisk the egg and shredded Mozzarella cheese together. If you do not have shredded Mozzarella cheese, you can use the shredder to shred your cheese, add the almond powder and baking powder to the bowl and whisk them until the mixture is consistent.
2. Then pour the mixture onto the waffle machine. Make sure you pour it to the center of the mixture will come out of the edges on closing the machine.

3. Close the machine and let the waffles cooking until golden brown. Then you can serve your tasty chaffle waffles.

Nutrition:

Calories: 170, Fat: 15g, Protein: 7g, Net Carbs: 2g

Keto Chaffle Topped with Salted Caramel Syrup

Preparation: 15 minutes

Cooking: 10 minutes

Servings: 2

Ingredients

- 1 egg
- ½ cup of Mozzarella cheese
- ¼ cup of cream
- 2 tbspn of collagen powder
- 1 ½ tbspn of almond flour
- 1 ½ tbspn of unsalted butter
- Pinch of salt
- ¾ tbspn of powdered erythritol
- Pinch of baking powder

Directions

1. Begin by Preheat nowing your waffle machine by switching it on and turning the heat to medium.

2. Whisk together the chaffle ingredients that include the egg, Mozzarella cheese, almond flour, and baking powder. Pour the mixture on the waffle machine.
3. Let it cooking until golden brown. You can make up to two chaffles with this method.
4. To make the caramel syrup, you will need to turn on the flame under a pan to medium heat Melt now the pan's unsalted butter.
5. Then turn the heat low and add collagen powder and erythritol to the pan and whisk them.
6. Gradually add the cream and Remove now from heat. Then add the salt and continue to whisk.
7. Pour the syrup onto the chaffle, and here you go.

Nutrition:

Calories: 75, Fat: 7g, Protein: 1g, Net Carbs: 3g

Keto Chaffle Bacon Sandwich

Preparation: 15 minutes

Cooking: 10 minutes

Servings: 2

Ingredients

- 1 egg
- ½ cup of shredded Mozzarella cheese
- 2 Tbspn of coconut flour
- 2 strips of pork or beef bacon
- 1 slice of any type of cheese
- 2 tbspn of coconut oil

Directions

1. To make the chaffle, you will follow the typical recipe for making a chaffle. Start by warming your waffle machine to medium heat.
2. In a bowl, beat 1 egg, ½ cup of Mozzarella cheese, and almond flour.
3. Pour the mixture on the waffle machine. Let it cooking until it is golden brown. Then Remove now in a plate.

4. Warm coconut oil in a pan over medium heat.
5. Then place the bacon strips in the pan.
6. Cooking until crispy over medium heat.
7. Assemble the bacon and cheese on the chaffle.

Nutrition:

Calories: 225, Fat: 19g, Protein: 8g, Net Carbs: 3g

Crispy Zucchini Chaffle

Preparation: 15 minutes

Cooking: 5 minutes

Servings: 2

Ingredients

- 2 eggs
- 1 fresh zucchini
- 1 cup of shredded or grated cheddar cheese
- 2 pinches of salt
- 1 tbspn of onion (chopped)
- 1 clove of garlic

Directions

1. Start by Preheat nowing your waffle maker to medium heat. The best way to make a chaffle is to make it with layering. Start by dicing onions and mashing the garlic. Then use the grater to grate the zucchini. Then, take a bowl, add 2 eggs, and add the grated zucchini to the bowl.
2. Also, add the onions, salt, and garlic for extra flavor. You can also add other herbs to give your chaffle a

crispy more flavor. Then sprinkle ½ cup of cheese on top of the waffle machine.

3. Add the mixture from the bowl to the waffle machine. Add the remaining cheese on top of the waffle machine and close the waffle machine. Make sure the waffle cooking for about 3 to 5 minutes until it turns golden brown.
4. By the layering method, you will achieve the perfect crisp. Take out your zucchini chaffles and serve them hot and fresh.

Nutrition:

Calories: 100, Fat: 8.5g, Protein: 5.5g, Net Carbs: 0.5g

Peanut Butter Chaffle

Preparation: 15 min

Cooking: 10 min

Servings: 2

Ingredients

- 1 egg
- ½ cup of cheddar cheese
- 2 tbsps of peanut butter
- Few drops of vanilla extract

Directions

1. Take a grater and grate some cheddar cheese. Add one egg, cheddar cheese, 2 tbsps of peanut butter, and a few drops of vanilla extract. Beat these ingredients together until the batter is consistent enough.
2. Then sprinkle some shredded cheese as a base on your waffle maker. Pour the mixture on top of the waffle machine.
3. Sprinkle more cheese on top of the mixture and close the waffle machine. Ensure that the waffle is cooked

thoroughly for about a few minutes until they are golden brown. Then Remove now it and enjoy your deliciously cooked chaffles.

Nutrition:

Calories: 150, Fat: 10g, Protein: 16g, Net Carbs: 0.5g

Breakfast Chaffles With Berries

Preparation: 5 Min

Cooking: 5 Min

Servings: 4

Ingredients

Chaffle:

- 1 Cup Egg Whites
- 1 cup cheddar cheese, shredded
- ¼ cup almond flour
- ¼ cup heavy cream

Topping:

- 4 Oz. Raspberries
- 4 Oz. Strawberries.
- 1 Oz. Keto Chocolate Flakes
- 1 Oz. Feta Cheese.

Directions

1. Preheat now your square waffle maker and grease with cooking spray.
2. Beat egg white in a tiny bowl with flour.

3. Add shredded cheese to the egg whites and flour mixture and mix well.
4. Add cream and cheese to the egg mixture.
5. Pour Chaffles batter in a waffle maker and close the lid.
6. Cooking chaffles for about 4 minutes until crispy and brown.
7. Carefully Remove now chaffles from the maker.
8. Serve with berries, cheese, and chocolate on top.
9. Enjoy!

Nutrition:

Calories: 145, Fat: 12.5g, Protein: 5g, Net Carbs: 2g

Chaffle Breakfast Bowl

Preparation: 10 Min

Cooking: 5 Min

Servings: 2

Ingredients

Chaffle:

- 1 Egg
- 1/2 cup cheddar cheese shredded
- pinch of Italian seasoning
- 1 tbsp. pizza sauce

Topping:

- 1/2 Avocado Sliced
- 2 Eggs Boiled
- 1 Tomato, Halves
- 4 Oz. Fresh Spinach Leaves

Directions

1. Preheat now your waffle maker and grease with cooking spray.

2. Crack an egg in a tiny bowl and beat with Italian seasoning and pizza sauce.
3. Add shredded cheese to the egg and spices mixture.
4. Pour 1 tbsp. shredded cheese in a waffle maker and cooking for 30 sec.
5. Pour Chaffles batter in your waffle maker and close the lid.
6. Cooking chaffles for about 4 minutes until crispy and brown.
7. Carefully Remove now chaffles from the maker.
8. Serve on the spinach bed with boil egg, avocado slice, and tomatoes.
9. Enjoy!

Nutrition:

Calories: 75, Fat: 6g, Protein: 2.5g, Net Carbs: 2g

Chaffles With Sausage

Preparation: 5 Min

Cooking: 10 Min

Servings: 2

Ingredients

Chaffle:

- 1/2 cup cheddar cheese
- 1/2 tsp. baking powder
- 1/4 cup egg whites
- 2 tsp. pumpkin spice

Topping:

- 1 egg, whole
- 2 chicken sausage
- 2 slice bacon
- salt and pepper to taste
- 1 tsp. avocado oil

Directions

1. Mix all the chaffle ingredients in a bowl.
2. Allow batter to sit while waffle iron warms.

3. Spray waffle iron with nonstick spray.
4. Pour batter in your waffle maker and cooking according to the manufacturer's **Directions**.
5. Meanwhile, heat oil in a pan and fry the egg, according to your choice and transfer it to a plate.
6. In the same pan, fry bacon slice and sausage on medium heat for about 2-3 minutes until cooked.
7. Once chaffles are cooked thoroughly, Remove now them from the maker.
8. Serve with fried egg, bacon slice, sausages and enjoy!

Nutrition:

Calories: 319, Fat: 24 g, Net Carbohydrates: 1 g, Protein: 25 g

Mini-Breakfast Chaffles

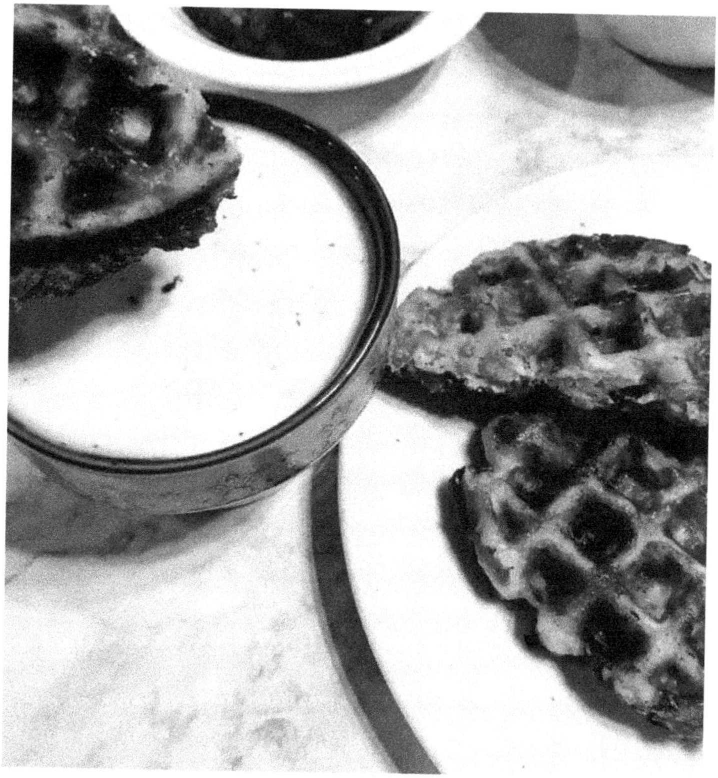

Preparation: 5 Min

Cooking: 15 Min

Servings: 3

Ingredients

Chaffle:

- 6 tsp. coconut flour
- 1 tsp. stevia
- 1/4 tsp. baking powder
- 2 eggs
- 3 oz. cream cheese
- 1/2. tsp. vanilla extract

Topping:

- 1 egg
- 6 slice bacon
- 2 oz. Raspberries for topping
- 2 oz. Blueberries for topping
- 2 oz. Strawberries for topping

Directions

1. Heat up your square waffle maker and grease with cooking spray.
2. Mix coconut flour, stevia, egg, baking powder, cheese and vanilla in mixing bowl.
3. Pour ½ of chaffles mixture in a waffle maker.
4. Close the lid and cooking the chaffles for about 3-5 minutes.

5. Meanwhile, fry bacon slices in pan on medium heat for about 2-3 minutes until cooked and transfer them to plate.
6. In the same pan, fry eggs one by one in the bacon's leftover grease.
7. Once chaffles are cooked, carefully transfer them to plate.
8. Serve with fried eggs and bacon slice and berries on top.
9. Enjoy!

Nutrition:

Protein: 16% 75 kcal, Fat: 75% 346 kcal, Carbohydrates: 9% 41 kcal

Coconut Chaffle

Preparation: 5 Min

Cooking: 5 Min

Servings: 2

Ingredients

- 1 egg
- 1 oz. cream cheese,
- 1 oz. cheddar cheese
- 2 tbsps. coconut flour
- 1 tsp. stevia
- 1 tbsp. coconut oil, Melt nowed
- 1/2 tsp. coconut extract
- 2 eggs, soft boil for serving

Directions

1. Heat you waffle maker and grease with cooking spray.
2. Mix all chaffles ingredients in a bowl.
3. Pour chaffle batter in a Preheat nowed waffle maker.
4. Close the lid.

5. Cooking chaffles for about 2-3 minutes until golden brown.
6. Serve with boil egg and enjoy!

Nutrition:

Protein: 21% 32 kcal, Fat: % 117 kcal, Carbohydrates: 3% 4 kcal

Bagel Chaffles with Peanut Butter

Preparation: 5 minutes

Cooking: 10 minutes

Servings: 2

Ingredients

- Eggs: 1
- Mozzarella cheese: ½ cup shredded
- Coconut flour: 1 tsp.
- Everything Bagel seasoning: 1 tsp.

For the filling:

- Peanut butter: 3 tbsp.
- Butter: 1 tbsp.
- Powdered sweetener: 2 tbsp.

Directions

- Add all the chaffle ingredients in a bowl and whisk
- Preheat now your mini waffle iron if needed and grease it
- Cooking your mixture in the mini waffle iron for at least 4 minutes

- Make as many chaffles as you can
- Mix now the filling ingredients
- When chaffles cool down, spread peanut butter

Nutrition:

Calories: 423 kcal, Protein: 26.07 g, Fat: 29.87 g, Carbohydrates: 16.04 g, Sodium: 120 mg

Ground Cinnamon Bread

Preparation: 5 minutes

Cooking: 10 minutes

Servings: 2

Ingredients

- Egg: 1
- Mozzarella Cheese: ½ cup (shredded)
- Ginger: ½ tsp. ground
- Erythritol: 1 tsp. powdered
- Ground cinnamon: ½ tsp.
- Ground nutmeg: ¼ tsp.
- Ground cloves: 1/8 tsp.
- Almond flour: 2 tbsp.
- Baking powder: ½ tsp.

Directions

1. Mix all the ingredients well together
2. Pour a layer on a Preheat nowed waffle iron
3. Cooking the chaffle for around 5 minutes

4. Make as many chaffles as your mixture and waffle maker allow
5. Serve with your favorite topping

Nutrition:

Calories: 332 kcal, Protein: 26.27 g, Fat: 22.47 g, Carbohydrates: 5.16 g, Sodium: 799 mg

Mushroom Stuffed Chaffles

Preparation: 15 minutes

Cooking: 40 minutes

Servings: 2

Ingredients

For Chaffle:

- Egg: 2
- Mozzarella Cheese: ½ cup (shredded)
- Onion powder: ½ tsp.
- Garlic powder: ¼ tsp.
- Salt: ¼ tsp. or as per your taste
- Black pepper: ¼ tsp. or as per your taste
- Dried poultry seasoning: ½ tsp.

For Stuffing:

- Onion: 1 tiny diced
- Mushrooms: 4 oz.
- Celery stalks: 3
- Butter: 4 tbsp.
- Eggs: 3

Directions

1. Preheat now a mini waffle maker if needed and grease it
2. In a mixing bowl, add all the chaffle ingredients and mix now them well
3. Pour the mixture to the lower plate of your waffle maker and spread it evenly to cover the plate properly and close the lid
4. Cooking for at least 4 minutes to get the desired crunch
5. Remove now the chaffle from the heat and keep aside
6. Make as many chaffles as your mixture and waffle maker allow
7. Take a tiny frying pan and Melt now butter in it on medium-low heat
8. Sauté celery, onion, and mushrooms to make them soft
9. Take another bowl and tear chaffles down into minute pieces
10. Add the eggs and the veggies to it
11. Take a casserole dish, and add this new stuffing mixture to it
12. Bake it at 350 degrees for around 30 minutes and serve hot

Nutrition:

Calories: 704 kcal, Protein: 49.35 g, Fat: 50.3 g, Carbohydrates: 12.84 g, Sodium: 888 mg

Minty Mini Chaffles

Preparation: 5 minutes

Cooking: 10 minutes

Servings: 2

Ingredients

- Eggs: 2
- Mozzarella: 1 cup shredded
- Cream cheese: 2 tbsp.
- Mint: ¼ cup chopped
- Almond flour: 2 tbsp.
- Baking powder: ¾ tbsp.
- Water: 2 tbsp. (optional)

Directions

1. Preheat now your mini waffle iron if needed
2. Mix all the ingredients mentioned above in a bowl
3. Grease your waffle iron lightly
4. Cooking your mixture in the mini waffle iron for at least 4 minutes or till the desired crisp is achieved and serve hot

5. Make as many chaffles as your mixture and waffle maker allow

Nutrition:

Calories: 559 kcal, Protein: 28.03 g, Fat: 41.69 g, Carbohydrates: 21.03 g, Sodium: 463 mg

Creamy Cinnamon Chaffles

Preparation: 5 minutes

Cooking: 10 minutes

Servings: 2

Ingredients

- Eggs: 2
- Shredded mozzarella: 1 cup
- Cream cheese: 2 tbsp.
- Cinnamon powder: 1 tbsp.
- Almond flour: 2 tbsp.
- Baking powder: ¾ tbsp.
- Water: 2 tbsp. (optional)

Directions

1. Preheat now your mini waffle iron if needed
2. Mix all the ingredients mentioned above in a bowl
3. Grease your waffle iron lightly
4. Cooking your mixture in the mini waffle iron for at least 4 minutes or till the desired crisp is achieved and serve hot

5. Make as many chaffles as your mixture and waffle maker allow.

Nutrition:

Calories: 582 kcal, Protein: 33.93 g, Fat: 44.06 g, Carbohydrates: 12.09 g, Sodium: 664 mg

Jalapeno Grilled Cheese Bacon Chaffle

Preparation: 15 minutes

Cooking: 20 minutes

Servings: 2

Ingredients

- Egg: 2
- Mozzarella Cheese: 1 cup (shredded)
- Jalapenos: 2 sliced with seeds Remove nowd along with the skin
- Cream cheese: ½ cup
- Monterey jack: 2 slices
- Cheddar cheese: 2 slices
- Bacon: 4 slices cooking

Directions

1. Add over two tbsps of cream cheese to the half-cut jalapenos
2. Bake them for around 10 minutes and set aside
3. Preheat now a mini waffle maker if needed and grease it

4. In a mixing bowl, beat eggs and add Mozzarella cheese to them and mix well
5. Pour the mixture to the lower plate of your waffle maker and spread it evenly to cover the plate properly
6. Cooking for at least 4 minutes to get the desired crunch
7. Remove now the chaffle from the heat and keep aside for around one minute
8. Make as many chaffles as your mixture and waffle maker allow
9. Make a sandwich by placing a slice of Monterey Jack, a cheese slice, 2 bacon slices in between two chaffles and enjoy!

Nutrition:

Calories: 295 kcal, Protein: 11.23 g, Fat: 24.4 g, Carbohydrates: 10.68 g, Sodium: 110 mg

Monte Cristo Chaffle

Preparation: 5 minutes

Cooking: 10 minutes

Servings: 2

Ingredients

For Chaffle:

- Egg: 2
- Cream cheese: 2 tbsp.
- Vanilla extract: 1 tbsp.
- Almond flour: 2 tbsp.
- Heavy cream: 1 tsp.
- Cinnamon powder: 1 tsp.
- Swerve sweetener: 1 tbsp.

For Assembling:

- Cheese: 2 slices
- Ham: 2 slices
- Turkey: 2 slices

Directions

1. Preheat now a mini waffle maker if needed and grease it
2. In a mixing bowl, add all the chaffle ingredients and mix now them well
3. Pour the mixture to the lower plate of your waffle maker and spread it evenly to cover the plate properly
4. Cooking for at least 4 minutes to get the desired crunch
5. Remove now the chaffle from the heat and keep aside for around one minute
6. Make as many chaffles as your mixture and waffle maker allow
7. Serve with a cheese slice, a turkey, and a ham
8. You can also serve with any of your favorite low carb raspberry jam on top

Nutrition:

Calories: 351; Total Fat: 36g; Carbs: 5g; Net Carbs: 4g; Fiber: 1g;

Savory Chaffles Bacon & Jalapeno Chaffles

Cooking: 15 Minutes

Servings: 5

Ingredients

- 3 tbsps coconut flour
- 1 teaspn organic baking powder
- 1/4 teaspn salt
- 1/2 cup cream cheese, softened
- 3 large organic eggs
- 1 cup sharp Cheddar cheese, shredded
- 1 jalapeno pepper, seeded and chopped
- 3 cooked bacon slices, crumbled

Directions

1. Preheat now a mini waffle iron and then grease it.
2. Place the flour, baking powder and salt and mix well in a tiny bowl.
3. Place the cream cheese and beat in a large bowl until light and fluffy.

4. Add the eggs and Cheddar cheese and beat until well combined.
5. Add the flour mixture and beat until combined.
6. Fold in the jalapeno pepper.
7. Divide the mixture into 5 portions.
8. Place 1 portion of the mixture into Preheat nowed waffle iron and cook for about 5 minutes or until golden brown.
9. Repeat now with the remaining mixture.
10. Serve warm with the TOPPING of bacon pieces.

Nutrition:

Calories: 249, Net Carb: 2.99g, Fat: 20.3g, Saturated Fat: 5g, Carbohydrates:4.8g, Dietary Fiber: 1.9g, Sugar: 0.5g, Protein: 12.7g

3-Cheese Broccoli Chaffles

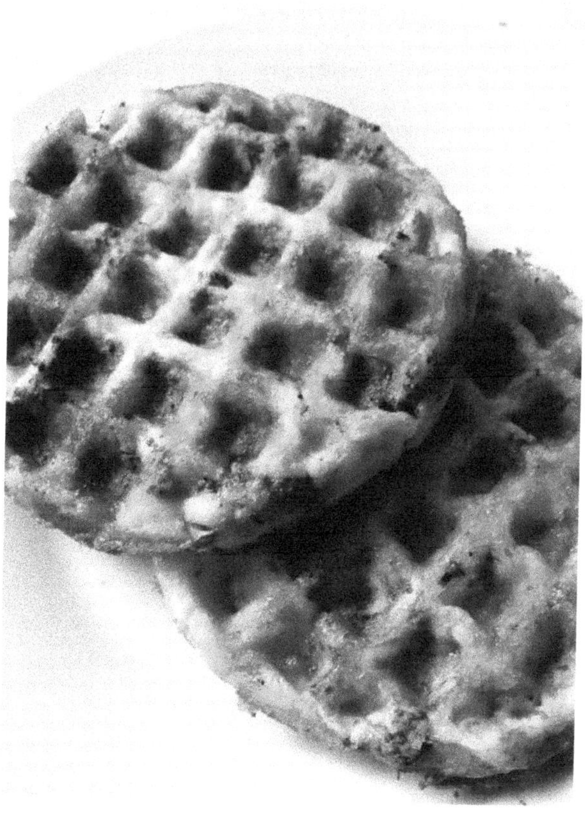

Cooking: 16 Minutes

Servings: 4

Ingredients

- 1/2 cup cooked broccoli, chopped finely

- 2 organic eggs, beaten
- 1/2 cup Cheddar cheese, shredded
- 1/2 cup Mozzarella cheese, shredded
- 2 tbsps Parmesan cheese, grated
- 1/2 teaspn onion powder

Directions

1. Preheat now a waffle iron and then grease it.
2. In a bowl, place all Ingredients and Mix well until well combined.
3. Place half of the mixture into Preheat nowed waffle iron and cook for about 4 minutes or until golden brown.
4. Repeat now with the remaining mixture.
5. Serve warm.

Nutrition:

Calories: 112, Net Carb: 1.2g, Fat: 8.1g, Saturated Fat: 4.3g, Carbohydrates:1.59g, Dietary Fiber: 0.3g, Sugar:0.5g, Protein: 8.

Bacon and Ham Chaffle

Cooking: 5 Minutes

Servings: 2

Ingredients

- 3 egg
- 1/2 cup grated Cheddar cheese
- 1 Tbsp almond flour
- 1/2 tsp baking powder

For the TOPPINGs:

- 4 strips cooked bacon
- 2 pieces Bibb lettuce
- 2 slices preferable ham
- 2 slices tomato

Directions:

1. Turn on waffle maker to heat and oil it with cooking spray.
2. Combine all chaffle components in a tiny bowl.
3. Add around 1/4 of total batter to waffle maker and spread to fill the edges. Close and cook for 4 minutes.
4. Remove now and let it cool on a rack.

5. Repeat for the second chaffle.
6. Top one chaffle with a tomato slice, a piece of lettuce, and bacon strips, then cover it with second chaffle.
7. Plate and enjoy.

Nutrition: Carbs: 5g ; Fat: 60 g ; Protein: 31 g ; Calories: 631

Ham & Cheddar Chaffles

Preparation: 15 minutes

Cooking: 28 minutes

Servings: 4

Ingredients

- 1 cup finely shredded parsnips, steamed
- 8 oz. ham, diced
- 2 eggs, beaten
- 1 ½ cups finely grated cheddar cheese
- ½ tsp. garlic powder
- 2 tbsp. chopped fresh parsley leaves
- ¼ tsp. smoked paprika
- ½ tsp. dried thyme
- Salt and freshly ground black pepper to taste

Directions

1. Preheat now the waffle iron.
2. In a bowl, mix all the ingredients.
3. Open the iron, lightly grease with cooking spray and pour in a quarter of the mixture.

4. Close the iron and cooking until crispy, 7 minutes.
5. Remove now the chaffle onto a plate and set aside.
6. Make three more chaffles using the remaining mixture.
7. Serve afterward.

Nutrition:

Calories: 99 Cal, Total Fat: 8 g, Saturated Fat: 0 g, Cholesterol: 0 mg, Sodium: 0 mg, Total Carbs: 4 g

Gruyere and Chives Chaffles

Preparation: 15 minutes

Cooking: 14 minutes

Servings: 2

Ingredients

- 2 eggs, beaten
- 1 cup finely grated Gruyere cheese
- 2 tbsp. finely grated cheddar cheese
- 1/8 tsp. freshly ground black pepper
- 3 tbsp. minced fresh chives + more for garnishing
- 2 sunshine fried eggs for topping

Directions

1. Preheat now the waffle iron.
2. In a bowl, mix now the eggs, cheeses, black pepper, and chives.
3. Open the iron and pour in half of the mixture.
4. Close the iron and cooking until brown and crispy, 7 minutes.
5. Remove now the chaffle onto a plate and set aside.
6. Make another chaffle using the remaining mixture.

7. Top each chaffle with one fried egg each, garnish with the chives and serve.

Nutrition:

Calories: 99 Cal, Total Fat: 8 g, Saturated Fat: 0 g, Cholesterol: 0 mg, Sodium: 0 mg, Total Carbs: 4 g

Hot Chocolate in Breakfast Chaffle

Preparation: 10 minutes

Cooking: 14 minutes

Servings: 2

Ingredients

- 1 egg, beaten
- 2 tbsp almond flour
- 1 tbsp unsweetened cocoa powder
- 2 tbsp cream cheese, softened
- ¼ cup finely grated Monterey Jack cheese
- 2 tbsp sugar-free maple syrup
- 1 tsp vanilla extract

Directions

1. Preheat now the waffle iron.
2. In a bowl, mix all the ingredients.
3. Open the iron, lightly grease with cooking spray and pour in half of the mixture.
4. Close the iron and cook until crispy, 7 minutes.
5. Remove now the chaffle onto a plate and set aside.

6. Pour the remaining batter in the iron and make the second chaffle.
7. Allow cooling and serve afterward.

Nutrition:

Calories: 99 Cal, Total Fat: 8 g, Saturated Fat: 0 g, Cholesterol: 0 mg, Sodium: 0 mg, Total Carbs: 2 g

Mini Breakfast Chaffle

Preparation: 10 minutes

Cooking: 15 Minutes

Servings: 3

Ingredients

- 6 tsp coconut flour
- 1 tsp stevia
- 1/4 tsp baking powder
- 2 eggs
- 3 oz. cream cheese
- 1/2. tsp vanilla extract

Topping:

- 1 egg
- 6 slice bacon
- 2 oz. Raspberries for topping
- 2 oz. Blueberries for topping
- 2 oz. Strawberries for topping

Directions

1. Heat up your square waffle maker and grease with cooking spray.
2. Mix coconut flour, stevia, egg, baking powder, cheese and vanilla in mixing bowl.
3. Pour ½ of chaffles mixture in a waffle maker.
4. Close the lid and cook the chaffles for about 3-5 minutes Utes.
5. Meanwhile, fry bacon slices in pan on medium heat for about 2-3 minutes Utes until cooked and transfer them to plate.
6. In the same pan, fry eggs one by one in the bacon's leftover grease.
7. Once chaffles are cooked, carefully transfer them to plate.
8. Serve with fried eggs and bacon slice and berries on top.
9. Enjoy!

Nutrition:

Calories: 480, Fat: 30 g, Net Carbohydrates: 4 g, Protein: 45 g

Chaffles With Egg & Asparagus

Preparation: 10 minutes

Cooking: 10 Minutes

Servings: 1

Ingredients

- 1 egg
- 1/4 cup cheddar cheese
- 2 tbsps. almond flour
- ½ tsp. baking powder

<u>Topping:</u>

- 1 egg
- 4-5 stalks asparagus
- 1 tsp avocado oil

Directions

1. Preheat now waffle maker to medium-high heat.
2. Whisk together egg, mozzarella cheese, almond flour, and baking powder

3. Pour chaffles mixture into the center of the waffle iron. Close your waffle maker and let cook for 5 minutes Utes or until waffle is golden brown and set.
4. Remove now chaffles from your waffle maker and serve.
5. Meanwhile, heat oil in a nonstick pan.
6. Once the pan is hot, fry asparagus for about 4-5 minutes Utes until golden brown.
7. Poach the egg in boil water for about 2-3 minutes Utes.
8. Once chaffles are cooked, Remove now from the maker.
9. Serve chaffles with the poached egg and asparagus.

Nutrition:

Calories: 843, Total Fat: 65g, Saturated Fat: 14g, Protein: 59g, Cholesterol: 156mg, Carbohydrates: 6g, Fiber: 1g, Net Carbs: 5g

Peanut Butter Cup Chaffles

Preparation: 5 minutes

Cooking: 15 minutes

Servings: 1

Ingredients

For the chaffle:

- Eggs: 1
- Mozzarella cheese: ½ cup shredded
- Cocoa powder: 2 tbsp.
- Espresso powder: ¼ tsp.
- Sugar free chocolate chips: 1 tbsp.

For the filling:

- Peanut butter: 3 tbsp.
- Butter: 1 tbsp.
- Powdered sweetener: 2 tbsp.

Direction

1. Add all the chaffle ingredients in a bowl and whisk

2. Preheat now your mini waffle iron if needed and grease it
3. Cooking your mixture in the mini waffle iron for at least 4 minutes
4. Make two chaffles
5. Mix now the filling ingredients
6. When chaffles cool down, spread peanut butter on them to make a sandwich

Nutrition:

Calories: 448; Total Fat: 34g; Carbs: 17g; Net Carbs: 10g; Fiber: 7g; Protein: 24g

Chocolaty Chaffles

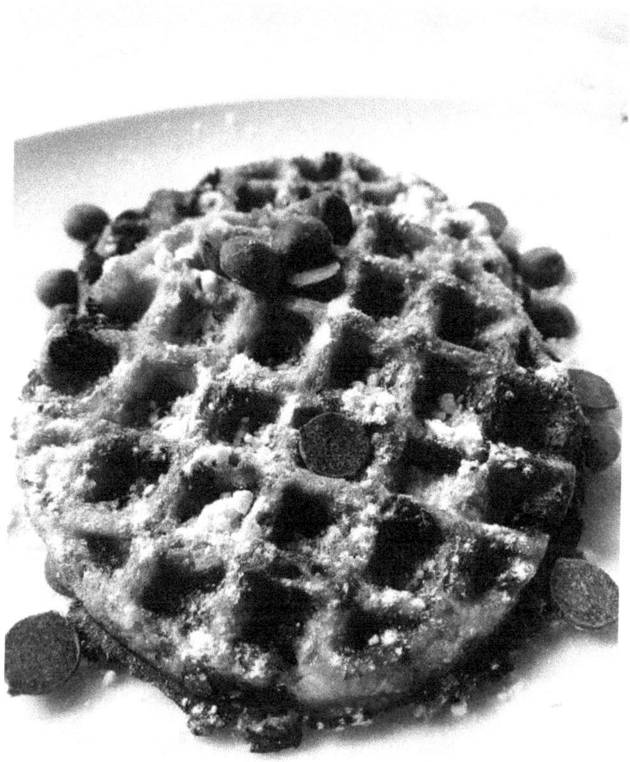

Preparation: 5 minutes

Cooking: 15 minutes

Servings: 1

Ingredients

- Eggs: 1
- Mozzarella cheese: ½ cup shredded
- Cocoa powder: 2 tbsp.
- Espresso powder: ¼ tsp.
- Sugar free chocolate chips: 1 tbsp.

Directions

1. Add all the chaffle ingredients in a bowl and whisk
2. Preheat now your mini waffle iron if needed and grease it
3. Cooking your mixture in the mini waffle iron for at least 4 minutes
4. Make as many chaffles as you can

Nutrition:

Calories: 258; Total Fat: 23g; Carbs: 12g; Net Carbs: 6g; Fiber: 6g; Protein: 5g

Bacon Chaffle Omelets

Cooking: 10 minutes | **Servings:** 2

Ingredients

- 2 slices bacon, raw
- 1egg
- 1 tsp maple extract, optional
- 1 tsp all spices

Directions

1. Put the bacon slices in a blender and tum it on.
2. Once ground up, add in the egg and all spices. Go on blending until liquefied.
3. Heat your waffle maker on the highest setting and spray with non-stick cooking spray.
4. Pour half the omelets into your waffle maker and cook for 5 minutes max.
5. Remove now the crispy omelet and repeat the same steps wit rest batter.
6. Enjoy warm

Nutrition:

Calories: 59 Kcal; Fats: 4.4 g: Carbs: 1 g: Protein: 5 g

Lightning Source UK Ltd.
Milton Keynes UK
UKHW052317100621
385265UK00008B/95

9 781802 6991